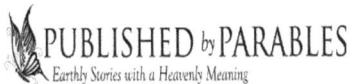

BY GOD'S GRACE
A TRUE LIVING TESTIMONY

JENNEFER PADDOCK

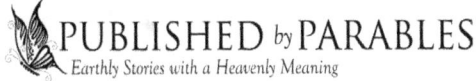
PUBLISHED by PARABLES
Earthly Stories with a Heavenly Meaning

By God's Grace: A True Living Testimony
Jennefer Paddock

Copyright © Jennefer Paddock

Published By Parables
July, 2018

All Rights Reserved. No part of this book may be reproduced or utilized in any form or by any means, electronic or mechanical, including photocopying, recording, or by any information storage and retrieval system, without permission in writing from the author.

Unless otherwise specified Scripture quotations are taken from the authorized version of the King James Bible.

    ISBN 978-1-945698-65-1
    Printed in the United States of America

Readers should be aware that Internet Web sites offered as citations and/or sources for further information may have been changed or disappeared between the time this was written and when it is read.

By God's Grace
A True Living Testimony

Jennefer Paddock

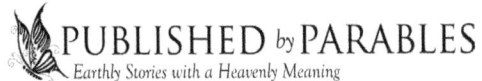
PUBLISHED by PARABLES
Earthly Stories with a Heavenly Meaning

BY GOD'S GRACE: A TRUE LIVING TESTIMONY

Table of Contents

Table of Contents — 7
The Lord's Prayer — 8
Dedication — 9
About The Author — 10
Chapter 1: Growing Up As A Child — 11
Chapter 2: When It All Began — 19
Chapter 3: The Inspiration — 23
Chapter 4: Answered Prayers — 27
Chapter 5: That Very Special Day — 31
Chapter 6: Releasing The Pain and Torment — 35
Chapter 7: Breaking The Cycle — 41
Chapter 8: Getting Healthy — 45
Chapter 9: Believing In Yourself — 49
Chapter 10: The Victory: Becoming a Survivor — 53
Poem Section — 57
Song Lyrics Section — 67

The Lord's Prayer
Matthew 6:9-13 (Life Application Study Bible/NLT)

"Our Father in heaven,
May your name be kept holy.
May your kingdom come soon.
May your will be done on earth,
As it is in heaven.
Give us today the food we need,
and forgive us our sins,
as we have forgiven those who sin against us.
And don't let us yield to temptation,
but rescue us from the evil one."

DEDICATION

This book is dedicated to God, first and foremost because He is using my story to be a blessing to those who are broken and lost. Thank you God for calling me into ministry.

Also, this book is dedicated to those that made this happen by inspiring me to be the best that I can be, and the encouragement I needed. Thank you for your support.

A special thank you goes out to my special friend, Darin "Tadpole" Davis for allowing God to work through you when you sent me all those encouraging words.

A special thank you goes out to the Woo-Hoo lady, who sows seeds of acceptance. Thank you for allowing God to work through you to be a blessing to others.

About The Author

I am a blessed, mother of three beautiful children. I have a passion for helping others and reaching to the lost. God is my rock, salvation, and my everything. I grew up as a broken girl, but now I have a Great and Mighty Healer who has made me new. I am very strong in my faith, and I believe that anyone can heal from their burdens, turmoil, disasters, and pain. God has blessed me in so many ways that seemed unimaginable. Anything is possible if you believe, and when you believe in yourself, you are half way there. Music has always been soothing to my soul, and the lyrics in the songs helped me to keep my faith, trust, and belief in God. I was called into ministry and By God's Grace, my journey has begun.

JENNEFER PADDOCK

Chapter 1-
Growing Up As a Child

    It all started when God blessed my parents on February 28, 1977. According to my parents, my birth was not planned, which is okay. Growing up as a little girl, I had a brother who was five years older than me, and my brother always terrorized his younger sister. Due to being the only girl, I grew up doing everything my brother and his friends would do; therefore, becoming a tom-boy. Growing up as a little girl, I looked up to my brother as if he was my hero. I remember having baby dolls, barbies, and stuffed animals; however, it was the matchbox cars, army men, and transformers that I wanted to play with.

    Growing up as a child, I grew up in a small town called Galesburg, Michigan. This town was so small that you could ride your bike to the store, lake, school, or anywhere you needed to go. There were busses, yellow cheese wagons as I always called them, that transported children to and from school; however, I walked to school most of the time. On days when I didn't walk to school, my friend's mom, Mrs. Lemon, picked me up on her bicycle. Mrs. Lemon was a bus driver, and there were times that I would ride the bus in order to clean up the bus. To this day, I have never seen Mrs. Lemon drive a car. I always see her walking, running, or riding her bike anywhere she needs to go.

    When I was about five years old, my parents began entering me into pageants. The very first pageant that I was entered in, I won "Little Miss Galesburg." Being as young as I was, I really did not have the excitement about winning as I do now as an adult. Waving at all the people at the parade, I remember the float being so pretty and full of flowers. The cool thing about riding the floats was that most of friends were on them too, along with Miss Galesburg. I got to throw candy out to the kids watching the parade. I can remember that after the parade was over, there was a day full of games, riding horses, dancing, singing, and prize drawings.

Throughout my younger years, I can remember all of the abuse that started shortly after winning my first pageant. I can always remember my dad coming home from work drunk, and all of the yelling and screaming between my mom and dad. Believe me, my dad, the monster, was never loving at all. He was always so abusive with his words, and he constantly yelled at me for hours. While my mom just watching, he would beat me with belts for hours, and he always made me cry. I can remember hiding under my bed just to avoid the beatings. My mom suffered abuse from the monster, as well as my brother. I do not remember my brother getting the beatings as much as I did. I grew up feeling that the reason I was constantly traumatized was because my parents didn't love or want me. I began growing up as a broken girl, just like the lyrics to the song "Broken Girl" by Matthew West says.

When I was six years old, I started attending a local church with my brother, where we went to VBS yearly. My brother and I never missed a Sunday until one day when I had a bicycle accident on the way to church. That morning, I remember begging the monster to take me to church in the car; however, he continued yelling at me, saying "I am not taking you to church in the car. I am taking you to church on the bike, and you will ride on the handle bars." Getting all dressed up and ready for church, it was time to get on the handle bars and head to church. Approaching the church and being one block away, my foot got caught in the fork of the front tire. The monster flat refused to stop the bike when my foot got caught, and he just kept peddling. What I remember the most is that the monster jerked my foot out of the front wheel, and left me there with my mom in the middle of the road because he was so mad that his bike was broke. To this day, I never understood why he was so mad about the bike because it was my money that I won from a pageant that bought the family bicycles. That accident prevented me from going to Sunday school and to church for half the year because I broke all the growth plates in my foot. I couldn't even go to school because I had to keep my foot elevated every day and go to the doctor's office every other day. I was broken because I could not go to the places where I had a break from the abuse.

At the age of nine, the monster told me and my brother that he was filing for a divorce. I didn't understand what all that meant so I asked him. His reply was " I am going to be moving out and leaving your mother. You will not see me every day, and I will be moving in with your grandma." I was crushed, devastated, and did not know what was going to happen. While my parents were going through the thing they call divorce, I remember having to talk to Child Protective Services every other day. They always came to school and pulled me out of class, and I was so embarrassed when I got back to class. I remember the people asking me so many questions that I did not understand. There was one day that they came to school because my brother slapped me so hard that he left a bruised handprint on my face. Once again, my mom just watched me get harmed by my brother, and he never got punished for it. At this moment in time, I began to feel that my brother did not want me around either because the one that I looked up to was now hurting me too. I constantly asked myself the questions "Why do they not love me? Why do they not want me? Why do they blame me?"

At the age of eleven, both parents remarried. Now I have two other parents that I wondered if they would love me or would they hurt me. For about a year or so, things were going great, until the monster was going through another divorce with my step-mom. Once again, I was devastated because I was loosing a little step-sister and a step-mom, whom I loved dearly. I was feeling that she did not love me either and that was why she was leaving too. Still today, I still can see the day when my step-mom came and moved all of her belongings out of the house and taking my little sister with her. After she left, the monster started becoming mean again but this time hitting me in the head. I had no one there to help me or protect me. The only thing that I was seeing was that no one wanted me and that no one loved me. Now I was being bounced back and forth between my mom and the monster's house. Being bounced back and forth, I always wondered if the monster would show up to get me, or would he be too busy with someone else. He always had a habit of not showing up to pick us up because he always had more important things to do than to be with his kids.

At the age of thirteen, my mom and step-dad made the executive decision to move to another state. Settling into another school and home, I had to make friends all over again. After we relocated to another state, I started being sexually abused by my step-father. I remember being scared when it started because my mom was not around when it started. My mom was temporarily gone for about 6 months to take care of personal business. Once my mom left, I was left in the hands of my step-dad and with my little step-brother. I always kept in the back of my mind if my mom would just watch that too, or would she stop it. So now, I started having to become a grown up at a early age. I had to do all the cooking, the cleaning, the laundry, yard work, caring after my little brother, at the same time the sexual abuse began. Once again, I had no one around to help me, protect me, or be there for me. The feeling of rejection started sinking in because the monster had left me there too. To me, the monster didn't try to get me away from the situations I was in. I was having to deal with all of this while attend school. I remember not being able to concentrate at school because my mind stayed so occupied. Not being able to concentrate at school, I begged the monster to come and get me; however, he never showed. All that I knew was that there was no way that I was going to be able to tell anyone what was happening to me because I was ashamed and afraid of what would happen. There was a time when I even ran away just to get away from all the abuse, but the cops made me go back home.

At the age of fifteen, I got the courage to start telling someone about what was going on at home. My friend, Libby, took me to the guidance counselor at school. Because I lived in another state from the monster, my counselor gave me a written assignment to do. My written assignment was to write the judge on the case a letter, and she mailed it to the court for me. I was 600 miles away from the judge so I had to write him a letter in order for him to read it. I was able to start talking to Child Protective Services, as well as the judge. While all this was going on, I was being told what to say and what not to say. Out of fear, I would listen to my abuser and do exactly what he told me to say. I was always being told that my dad did not love me, my dad did not want me, and I was always kept from my dad. My mom kept me from talking to my dad, and she would not even let me see my dad.

The cool thing about the judge was that because I was a child, I was able to talk to the judge in the judge's chambers. I felt safe because neither my mom or the monster was in the judge's chambers with me so no one knew what I was telling the judge. I was already being threatened with certain family in my life being killed. For the first time ever, I felt safe enough to tell someone what was going on at home. By me telling the judge and Child Protective Services what was going on I was able to break free from the abuse being inflicted by my step-dad, and I was able to move back to the monster's house. It took me being brave in order to get away from my sexual abuser. I knew that when I gained the courage to speak, I was able to break free from the abuse. After I was able to get away from my sexual abuser, I was able to tell my dad everything that had been going on, and I started to feel better by letting the truth out.

When I got back to my dad's house, I had a new step-mom who tried helping me along the way. My step-mom was very strict and always wanted me to do everything her way, and if I didn't then she would be mean to me too. During the summer, I heard that the marching band was looking for color guards, so I joined the marching band. I loved being in the marching band and going to competitions as well. My step-mom pushed me hard to excel in school to the point that when I made a D on a test in history class, she grounded me and made me study for two hours a night. I was not able to talk on the phone, see my friends, or go out and do anything with my friends. From that moment on, I never got a D on another test again, matter of fact, I made all A's on my history exams. Things were going well for me being back in Michigan, where I felt safe until Christmas break when I had to go visit my mom.

When I got to my mom's house for Christmas break, I had every intention of packing up my pageant trophies, and my personal belongings in an empty suitcase that I brought down with me. My mom has always been the nosy type, and when she looked in my suitcase, she seen all the tissue paper I had put in it to wrap up my trophies. That made my mom so mad that she instructed me to go for a walk. While I was on my walk, she called my dad and started another war with him and my step-mom. After the long, dreadful week with my mom and step-dad, I was taken back to my dad's house. When I arrived back to my dad's house, my step-mom was so cold to me, along with my dad. My step-mom called me everything but a white woman, and told me to pack up my things and threw me out of the house. My dad did not do anything to stop her, in fact, he supported her. Once again, I was tormented with the feelings of not being loved, not feeling wanted, feeling rejected and feeling unworthy of love. The question was "Where am I going to go now." My dad called up my mom while she was still in town and told her to come and pick me up. I was devasted, broken, and hurt because I was forced to go back to a place I did not want to be. The most depressing part was that I had to leave behind my boyfriend, whom I made plans to marry after graduation.

When I got back to Tennessee with my mom, the abuse started back up again, except this time, my step-dad was being very mean to my mom as well. My mom was abusing my step-brother, and I still can see the bruises that she left on his legs. The bruises were so bad, that I was able to see them through his long johns. No one was protecting me or my step-brother. All I knew was that I had to do whatever I had to do to make it until I was eighteen in order to go back to Michigan to marry my love. I started working as a way to cope with the abuse, stress, and rejection. I always made sure that I cared after my little brother, who suffered the abuse too. When I tried to tell my step-dad about the bruises, he chose not to listen. Once again, I became this broken girl watching her step-brother becoming a broken boy who later on got into drugs as a way to cope with the pain. Once again, I became alone with no one to help me, protect me, save me, love me, nurture me, or guide me. I finished high school hiding behind the broken girl.

After graduation, I went back to Michigan in order to marry my love; however, when I arrived I found out that he was married to someone else. Shattered, torn, and broken once again. I tried making my way in Michigan; however, I was all alone up there. I had a few friends that I hung out with, but my friends were busy with there own lives. I did not spend much time with my family either, so I felt very lonely. I kept my hope, faith, and trust in the one person who made promises to me that he never kept. For several months, I tried finding my way in Michigan, but didn't succeed. Feeling like a failure, I decided to move back to the Great Smokey Mountains to start my life over. From that moment on I realized that I could not depend on others or trust them; therefore, remaining alone.

BY GOD'S GRACE: A TRUE LIVING TESTIMONY

Chapter 2- When It All Began

The inspiration began on Wednesday January 24th, 2001 when God took control of my life. Drinking my morning cup of coffee, I was thinking about life's direction. As I was sitting in the reclining chair, I felt a presence of angels. Feeling the presence of angels, cold chills began running up and down my spine, then throughout my body. I remember my fingers feeling frozen, but they were warm to the touch. At first, I did not know what was happening to me until I heard God speaking to me saying, "You are a Child of God, and I sent my Son to be your guide through life. In order to reach me, you must go through my Son first." I had been to church as a child, but I never had this type of experience before. When I was a little child, I had asked Jesus to come into my heart; however, I did not exactly know what it truly meant at a very young age. As I became older, I knew that what was happening was God was touching my heart.

Knowing God had touched me, my heart was filled with warmth and tears strolled down my face. The tears were joyful tears, not tears of sadness or sorrow. Feeling deeply loved, burdens that had been carried for years were lifted. I can remember feeling fifty pounds lighter and feeling so relieved. Up until God touched me, I felt all alone, with no one around to love and care for me. It seemed as though the ones in my life loving me were only hurting and destroying me. Feeling destroyed, I always felt as if I was at rock bottom, with no way up. During the eye of the storms, along life's journey, God rescued me. I will admit, I had my fair share of faults, and I never felt forgiven of my sins and faults. When God rescued me, I felt forgiven for the first time ever. Nothing compares to the feeling of joy I had, for I was beginning the journey that God had for me.

Throughout the years, I still continued to feel lost in the eye of the storm, with nowhere to turn. I felt like no matter how hard I tried, I always stayed at rock bottom. Every direction I took in life always ended up at a dead end. I would constantly take the advice from others; however, I was taking advice from all the wrong people. I felt as if I was never good enough at anything I did, and I felt as if I would never be accepted or loved for who I was. Carrying negative labels given by others, I always hid behind who God created me to be because I did not know my purpose in life. For so long, I felt as if my purpose was to always be tormented and torn; thus, preventing me to know what my purpose and calling was. Still unclear of my purpose, I continued to pray to God to show me what my purpose was and continued to ask God, "Why me?"

After many prayers, I met a friend who began to show me what love is, as well as what love is supposed to be. Being hesitant, I listened to everything my friend said about love, Jesus, and the Bible. I was at a point in my life where I did not understand anything my friend was saying. Being called a goat, I continued listening to my friend daily. Every day, my friend would tell me what scriptures to read and what to study. Every day and night, we would talk about the scriptures and pray. I remember asking myself, "Why is my friend doing this for me? What is he expecting in return?" The reality is, God instructed him to show me what love is and what love is supposed to be. Being trapped in the middle of life's trials and tribulations, I was not able to see God's blessing or understanding when I met my friend. It was not until I decided to move a few states away before I began to understand what my friend was telling me.

Making the decision to move states away was a difficult decision because my son was about to graduate high school and attend college. After many conversations with my son, we agreed that it was ok to move and take the better job. I struggled week to week trying to provide for my son and I, so accepting the better job was an opportunity for advancement. I went back to where life began for me, my birth state. As time went on, I started realizing what my friend was telling me about love and letting others dictate my emotions. So many years I prayed for so many answers; however, I still never had the clear, true answers. I was beginning to think and feel that God was not listening to me or He was just choosing to ignore me. I often thought that God was maybe punishing me for something by not giving me the answers; although deep down inside I knew that was not the case.

Coming from a traumatic, abusive, childhood, I lacked the right type of parent love, nurture, and care. Due to the abuse at home, I ended up in foster care, where my aunt and uncle cared for my brother and I. I remember having to switch schools and make new friends all over again. If it wasn't for my family taking us in, we would have remained at the foster home. One night in the foster home was so scary, and I never forget what that experience was like. As I got older, I began to realize that all the pieces to the puzzle never added up. Growing up, I always looked at life as a puzzle, where I used the puzzle as life's direction. The problem I faced was that so many pieces were missing out of the puzzle.

Going back to my birth state is where God starting showing the answers to so many questions I have had for so long. When I moved back to my birth state, I moved to a house which was in the same city as I grew up in. I grew up in a little town called Galesburg, Michigan, where you could walk or ride a bike to anywhere you needed to go. Moving back to Galesburg, I moved to a house that was five houses down from the house that contained so many haunting memories. Some memories were good, but for the most part, the memories continued to haunt me. I faced the haunting memories day after day, hour after hour, minute after minute, and second after second. Throughout life, I carried those haunting memories that came from the blue, broken home that was remodeled to look like a barn. Going through life, I always wanted to revisit that broken home so that I could face the memories and the hurt.

As each passing day went by, I was able to see the broken home without tears falling down from my face. There were times I still cried because of the pain and turmoil in the home; however, as time went on it was easier to deal with. One day, I ran into the owners of the home, and I learned that the house was up for sale by owner. I explained to the couple that I grew up in the home and would like to see it. True healing came when I was able to walk in the home, walk in every room, walk the property, and walk in the garage without falling apart. When I went back to that broken home, I was able to leave the haunting memories there and pick up from where I left off, at the age of fifteen. It was my heart's desire to revisit that home to pick up where I left off, when I left the home at the age of fifteen. Carrying the haunting memories with me, I was able to leave those memories behind. I had to leave the memories where they came from, and after I did that, my life's journey began. True healing took place when I confronted the haunting memories and leaving them behind me. That is when I began to realize that the past was destroying me from the inside out.

Chapter 3 – The Inspiration

After high school graduation in 1995, I was going to use my full-ride scholarship to attend college. Graduating in the top 15% of my graduating class, I knew that I could be anything that I wanted to be. At the point in my life, I had planned on becoming a police officer. When I graduated high school, I temporarily moved away from home and went and stayed with some family to figure out exactly what I wanted to do with my life. Still of unsure of life's direction at the time, I held off going to college. I decided to take some time out for me and figure things out. I worked at ice cream shops, fast food restaurants, and a doughnut shop until I figured out what to do next. I had many thoughts about joining the air force; however, I decided to not choose that path.

As years went on, I continued working until I had my first born child in 1996. I met a man whom I thought would be an everlasting relationship, but to my surprise, it ended. For several years, I just took care of my son and I until my second born child was born. I remember being in a place where I felt all alone without any help from anyone. I raised the boys on my own without help from their absent parent. Raising two small boys on my own, I started praying for a direction. I knew that eventually I was going to have to think about a career in order to provide for my children, and to give them a better life than what I had growing up. With many career choices, I was leaning towards becoming a lawyer; however, I decided against that and became a paralegal instead. I started out being a paralegal just to see if being a lawyer was what I wanted to really be. Once I realized the arguing that lawyers have to do, I decided that I would not become one because I do not like to argue. I started seeing the corruption that was involved in the judicial system, and that is when I decided to not pursue becoming a lawyer.

After a few years of being a paralegal, my boss passed away; thus changing career paths. From the law office, I went into the timeshare industry and prepared contracts for a while. One thing that I found out was that I am too active to sit behind a desk for 8-10 hours a day, so I advanced to a management position where I was able to walk around more. I continued working for the company for several years until I focused on my career and what career would best suit me. I decided that I would go back to school to obtain a degree in the medical field. I decided to go back to college and get a degree in medical assisting because I am so passionate about helping others. Besides, I knew that I would be on my feet most of the day, and I could help others as well. I remember asking myself, "Is this really what you are supposed to do? Am I sure that I want to rack up more student loans?"

Racking up more student loan debt, I finished up my medical assisting degree in a year and a half. When I completed the program, I started working in the medical field, where I became a part of patient care. My passion has always been helping others, so I fit right in. Eight years later, I get this feeling that I am supposed to be something else, so I started working on a therapist degree. Half way through the program, I decided to drop out because I realized that I did not need a degree or college education to help others. I remember telling myself "Jesus did not have a college education to help and save us. Jesus did not have to study and pass written tests to do what He has done for us. Jesus never expected payment for what He does for us." From this moment on, I started seeing my purpose. My purpose is to help others and to work for God and whatever He may have me do.

In 2001, God instructed me to start writing a book. I remember thinking there was no way that I could ever be a writer, and I asked myself what would I even write about. I never thought or dreamed that I would become a writer or illustrator, let alone having my books published. I even questioned God many times regarding being called to write. I tried convincing myself that I would not be able to write books, they will never get published, it might be a waste of my time, and others might judge me for what I do write. Even though I had those thoughts, I began working on my first book. The feeling I had was like none other because I realized writing is a beautiful art. I remember feeling nervous about how to start the book and what I was actually going to write on; however, writing became natural.

Growing up I used to write poems, songs, stories, and of course, papers for school. To me writing was therapeutic. I wrote the first few chapters of my first book and called a friend to read my book so far. I was a little nervous about what my friend might think or if my friend would be judgmental, and then I remembered that the Bible says in Matthew to judge not. Remembering that, I felt at ease. After reading the first portion of the book to my friend, my friend responded and said "That was so touching. To look at you a week ago, now look at you. You are on the right path, and your testimony could touch some lost soul." From then on, I knew that God had called me to be a writer. My writing did not just stop with writing a book. I started writing procedure manuals for offices, employee manuals, and employee handbooks.

Writing has always been my passion, and writing has always been therapeutic to me. Trials and tribulations had forced me to lock up my book until the day I could finish it. Every time I picked up the book to start writing, it seemed like something else came up that took me away from it. Over the years, I have heard pastors talking about obedience and if God has instructed you to do something then you need to be obedient. There was this one certain sermon where the pastor talked about writing, and if you have been instructed to write then you need to do so. I remember sitting in the church pew thinking to myself that God was talking directly to me. During this time God was laying on my heart to write a few other books; however, I was not finished with the first one yet. I remember thinking to myself that there was no way I was ever going to be able to write all these books that He wants me to write.

What I came to realize is that writing has always been easy

for me to do. The problem has always been that I carried all this torment, pain, anger, and hurt that prevented me from accomplishing what God has instructed me to do all along. I went through life doing things my way or what others wanted me to do. I was failing to realize that I was not doing what God wanted me to do; therefore, being disobedient to His will. It took me a long time and a lot of debt to figure out that I was not doing what God had instructed me to do all along; however, I am in a place and frame of mind that I can do what God instructs me to do. The joy that I have in my heart knowing that I am finally able to do what God has instructed me to do, despite everything that I have been through. God has truly answered so many prayers that I have had for so many years. All these years when I thought God was not listening, He has shown me that He was listening to me. Also, He has shown me the answers to everything I have prayed about for so long.

No matter what you go through in life, if God instructs you to do something, you need to be obedient. Looking back on it, I realize that I could have saved me some heartache if I was obedient to His will. God has a plan for you, just like he had for me. Cast all of your burdens down in order to listen to God.

Chapter 4- Answered Prayers

As I began growing into adulthood, things never added up quite the way as others portrayed it to be. The pieces to the puzzle never added up. A lot of times, I asked family members so many questions about answers that I had been looking for. Growing up, I had so many questions as to why I was made to feel the way I felt and why I was so mistreated. I constantly asked God why no one loved me, why no one cared for me, and why I was constantly mistreated. I always felt as if I was the black sheep, and I often thought that I was mistreated because I was not planned. Growing up, I was always told that my dad tried killing me when I was in my moms womb. She always told me that my dad threw her through a wall, almost killing me. For as long as I can remember, I always asked God to show me the truth.

When I decided to take a position in Michigan in 2015, God started answering so many questions that I asked answers for. From the moment when God starting showing me the answers, I had a better understanding of what I had went through and why I felt the way I felt. When I went back to Michigan, I was faced with finding out that the man I thought was my dad wasn't even my real dad. I became thankful that the monster was not my dad. That made a lot of sense to me considering my mom told me that my dad could not have anything to do with me until I was eighteen. I began to understand why I always felt like the black sheep because in a lot of ways I was. I began to see where exactly I came from and who my real family was. I had peace of mind knowing where I came from. I questioned God has to why the truth was kept from me for so long, and He showed me that my mom and real dad was ashamed, and that my real parents were hiding behind the lies. I prayed for guidance, and God led me to the one who knew the truth, and to the one that always had my back growing up. At this point in my life, it doesn't matter who my dad is or who my dad isn't, what matters the most is that God revealed the truth. The reality is I have a Heavenly Father that will always love me, will always accept me, and He will never harm me in anyway. Without Him, I have nothing.

Knowing the truth made a huge difference to me because I was trying to live the life that I had deserved to live so long ago. The life that God intended me to live was interfered with way too long. God carried me back to my roots in order to show me what I had asked for. In the meantime, I carried so much anger, pain, torment, hurt, and disgust against others that it prohibited me from seeing what I had asked to be shown. Once I found out the truth, I was able to start releasing the burdens that I had carried for so long. I was able to look at life with a new set of lenses, and I knew that I was not going to go backwards in life. I had no choice but to start looking forward, so I started letting go of the haunting past. Growing up I longed for healthy relationships, a healthy marriage, and for positive people around me. I always associated love with pain, so I looked at people's actions towards me to know if they truly cared and loved me or not. What I began realizing is that just because someone says they love you, they don't always.

One thing I prayed so hard for was a brand new start at life, and to have a life that I could have a daughter that I could be there for. Because my mom was never there for me, I chose to be the opposite of her. I felt like a failure in life and worthless mother because my daughter was taken away from me by her dad. Her dad took her away from me just like my mom had taken me away from my dad. I prayed for a new start with someone who truly loved me the way that Jesus loves me, and I prayed that I would have a loving, Godly family. God answered my prayer when I was able to be a God mother to a fifteen year old who was broken just like I was. I thank God that I met her because of my life's experiences, I was able to help her overcome many of her obstacles in life. Just like me, she felt alone with no one to listen to her or help. With that experience, God showed me that I was helping myself by helping another broken girl, and then I knew how to help my own daughter through her obstacles. I had to heal from my past in order to move forward in life. I could not move forward carrying all of the heavy burdens. Not only did God place a God daughter in my life, God started placing true, Godly people in my life.

Ever since I was fifteen, I prayed for my love to come back into my life. Him and I had plans of getting married in August of 1995; however, he ended up marrying someone else and starting a family of his own. I begged and pleaded with God to one day bring him back to me so that I could pick up the pieces where we had left off when I was fifteen. For three months straight, I prayed for God to send me a true friend to go out with me, to hold me when I needed to be held, to wipe my tears when I needed to cry, a shoulder to lean on when I needed to talk, and someone to show me the right type of love instead of the type of love that was full of pain. I prayed for my best friend back. January 1, 2016, God blessed me with my best friend, the one that I was in love with since I was fifteen. What I never knew was that he was in Michigan the whole time I was. Around the time I moved back to Michigan, his wife had asked him for a divorce. Then I began to understand why God carried me back to Michigan. God carried me back to Michigan to pick up where I left off at 15, and to be there for him while he was going through a divorce after a 23 year marriage.

My relationships that I had as an adult ended up in disaster. The relationships that I ended getting involved in were just like the relationships I grew up in, full of pain, hurt, and torment. I always prayed for a loving husband and a loving father to my children. God answered my prayers when He brought my best friend and love back into my life. When he waltzed back into my life, that is when I started to be shown how I was supposed to be treated, as well as being a positive role model to my children. It has been a rough, rocky road for us both because we both were bogged down with heavy burdens; however, we are still growing strong. I am so thankful that God put him back in my life because it showed me exactly what I have for him and what I held onto for so long.

I thank God each and every day for the answered prayers. One thing that I discovered throughout life was that I have always had someone with me no matter the situation. Every time I prayed for someone to be there for me, God showed me that I will always have a friend anytime I need one, and that is Jesus. God sent His only begotten Son to die on the cross for me so that I can have eternal life. Jesus died on the cross for my sins, as well as everyone else, so that I and we could have eternal life. That is amazing, and I will never walk alone because through my life, Jesus has always been beside me. I was too bogged down by heavy burdens that I was never able to truly see that. The day I started seeing that, I was given the admiration and inspiration to free myself of all the heavy burdens so that I could be the loving, Godly wife to a man who God will truly bless me with. My desire has been to let go of the past and the labels that came with it, in order to marry the Godly husband that God has chosen for me without bringing the baggage into the relationship. By the grace of God and His Son, I have been able to start ridding myself of the past in order to prepare myself for what God has in store for me next.

Chapter 5- That Very Special Day

In April 2016, I had the pleasure of showing someone what love is and what unconditional love is. When I love others, I love like Jesus loves me. I was hurt by someone who told me they loved me, but made a choice to hurt me by cheating on me. Now I was faced with someone who was in a dark area in his life, but more so the one that I carried so much love for began cheating on me to, just like he had done to his ex-wife. I had every intention to confront him with it and let him go; however, God had other plans. Because I was still dealing with the past and he was going through a divorce, my first instinct was to run away from the relationship that was being built. The night I had gotten there to confront him, he was trying to lie his way out of it; however, I made him confront the truth. Because I know that the truth will set you free, it was my desire to free him of the truth. Long story short, he cried for a few hours, while I held him while he released his tears. Just when I thought things were going great in my life, my feelings got hurt once again. I witnessed to him and had a heart felt, lengthy conversation about Jesus's love for us. What I had realized that I was now dealing with someone else who said they loved me, but their actions showed different. I had to forgive him in order to move forward. I knew that in order to be forgiven myself, I had to forgive.

For the first time in my life, I chose not to run away from the heartache. What I came to realize was that he was going through trials and tribulations of his own, and he was not on God's side.

When he was tempted by the Tempter, he fell into temptation. I bared witness to him about Jesus, His love for us, and God could help him. I explained the importance in getting involved in a local church or perhaps a bible study. From listening to him, I realized that he was never truly shown what love is. He had the concept of knowing what love was, but the love he had always been shown was conditional love. So now here are two broken people trying to conquer our past. Give glory to God for having me bare witness because he started attending church with me, and he started reading the bible. The moral of the story is that no matter what anyone goes through, Jesus never leaves or forsakes us. If I had not have stayed that night, I would have lost an opportunity to help someone in need.

On my way home, as I was crying from the heart break, I encountered two beautiful deer that was standing in the middle of the road. I was enthralled at the beauty of the deer, that I wasn't thinking about not hitting them. I had automatically assumed that they would see me and move out of the way. Meeting deer in the middle of the road is something I am not used to doing; therefore, I did not know what I was supposed to do. I prayed that no other car would meet us on the road because I knew someone was going to get hurt. There were two bucks with big antlers, and each deer had a set of big eyes that were looking straight at me. By this time I knew that I was going to hit one of the deer, total my car, and get hurt myself, but at the time that I slammed on my brakes, each deer ran on opposite sides of the road.

Once I got calmed down and got my heart rate back down to a normal speed, I told God I understood, and the deer was a symbolism of what God was trying to show me. After getting home in one piece, and getting a good nights rest, I was able to fully understand the message that God was trying to show. On April 16, 2016, I asked God to take my whole heart, hold on to, mend it, make it new, and when the time was right, give it to the one that He has chosen to have it. For the first time ever, I felt lighter because when I asked God to take my heart and mend it, He took all the burdens carried for so long. God used the deer to show me that He had been there all along.

What I came to realize is that I had always looked for love

in all the wrong places. I failed to turn to God in anything I did. I knew that I had to mend my heart and free myself of 38 years of pain, hurt, anger, and torture, in order to have a healthy relationship. Instead of letting God drive the ship, I was always the driver. Then I starting realizing that the reason why I chose the relationships I did was because I was never shown any different growing up. What I came to realize was that God and His Begotten Son were the ones that would never hurt me in anyway, and they would always love me for who I am. It has been my heart's desire to love like Jesus, and when people encounter me they see the love of Jesus within me. I have had Jesus for a long time, but I never asked God to take my heart and hold it. That was the only way I was going to be able to heal. The cool part about it is that God does not ridicule you for what you have gone through.

What God showed me was that the reason why I was mistreated growing up was because my parents had been mistreated during their childhood and they never dealt with the past. To this day, they cling on to the past and they live in the past. Life is so simple and easy when you do not live in the past. It was not easy letting go and letting God, but I figured that I had nothing else to lose. Now what I have can never be taken away from me. I learned that I also lacked a close, personal relationship with God. Throughout life, every time I tried to draw near to God, the enemy got involved and pulled me away. These are all things that I was never truly shown by my parents; therefore, I lacked the understanding I needed.

Despite it all, I made God my everything. My Heavenly Father carries me through everything I go through in life, and He allows me to share my story with others in hopes that they will draw near to Him. It is all about the climb, and I am climbing uphill, not falling downhill. Once I made God my everything, He started showing me so much, and He continues to show me things. What I know is that God was there through everything that I went through, what I go through, and what I continue to go through. All along, what God wanted me to do was to draw near to Him so that He could show me a better way. If He can do this for me, I know that He will do this for everyone. Now, I commit everything I do, and I put all my trust in Him just like the bible says in Psalms 37:5-7

"Commit everything you do in the Lord.
Trust Him, and He will help you.
He will make your innocence radiate like the dawn,
And the justice of your cause will shine like the noonday sun.
Be still in the presence of the Lord,
And wait patiently for Him to act.
Don't worry about evil people who prosper
Or fret about their wicked schemes." (Life Application Study Bible)

God promises to love us when we need to be loved. God is our physician when we are ill and are in the need of healing. God is our army when we go to war, and He is our shield. When life rains down upon us, God is our umbrella. When we get weary, He is our rock and refuge. When we are drained, God is our strength. When no one else will listen to us, God is our voice. When no one will listen, God lends us His ear. When we feel pain, He is our comfort. When we are in darkness and under duress, God is our sunshine and hero. When you are frightened, God reaches His hand to hold us. When questions arise, God is our answer. God is our inspiration to overcome any obstacles that we face each and every day. It is God that gives us the admiration to remove the labels that holds us in bondage.

Chapter 6- Releasing the Pain and Torment

Throughout life, I carried so much pain and torment, along with the labels given by others. What was happening was, I was holding on to the deep, dark past; thus, causing me to carry the hurtful emotions and negative labels. So many times I tried laying the emotions and labels at Jesus's feet; however, I picked them back up to carry. Because I chose to carry the emotions and labels, I remained heavily burdened, as well as, being shackled by chains. Being shackled by chains, I stayed in complete conflict; therefore, never knowing where life would lead me.

Ever since I can remember, I always heard the words, "You are not good enough, you will never succeed in life, it is all your fault, you have done this to yourself, you will never be accepted, and you will never be happy." I was always told that I was a complete failure, and I was the one to always blame for others' wrongdoings. These were all words spoken to me by my abusers. Matter of fact, my last abuser looked me straight in the eye and said "I don't care." Suffering from abuse for so long, I began to believe the lies and comments from others. It was to the point in my life when I heard something positive, then I ran the other direction because I figured that they would drag me down too. When you hear those comments day after day, you begin to believe them. Believing all those comments for so long, my mind became manipulated in thinking that I was not worthy of love, joy, peace, kindness, and happiness.

Having a manipulated mind, I believed all the lies that everyone said. I chose all the wrong people to be around because I did not know any better. I spent most of my life looking for acceptance; therefore, I did my best to please others. I thought that if I pleased others, then I was accepted. Lacking the proper love, care, and nurture, I sought anyone that would show me love. I was always on my own because no one was ever there for me to listen. The abuse caused me to grow up rapidly, becoming a young lady at a very early age. I went through life feeling that everything was my fault; therefore, isolating myself from others and accepting all the wrong things. I was not able to see any other way because my abusers kept me bonded my chains.

As I grew older, I started realizing that it is not my fault, and I do not have to carry the blame anymore. Once I started to understand that it was not my fault, then I was able to start overcoming the negative comments from others. If it was up to my abusers, I would continue to believe that everything was my fault. Looking back on it now, if I would have had the right guidance early on, things in my life would have been so much different. No matter what I was believing or thinking, Jesus was always there, walking right beside me. I was never able to fully understand that I was truly never alone until I stopped blaming myself. The relief I have now knowing that I was truly never alone, helps me better cope with what I have had to cope with. It was almost like, no one ever wanted me to know that I had a personal Savior that would never leave my side.

When I stopped blaming myself, I was able to start talking about the abuse. One thing that a spiritual friend always told me was "The truth will always set you free, and all's that you ever need is love. When you have love, then you have everything." The love that my spiritual friend was meaning was the love of Jesus. What I started to understand and realize was that Jesus's love for me was what I needed in order to free myself of the pain and torture carried for so long. Truly knowing God's love for me, I started feeling accepted. What I come to know is, I looked for acceptance in all the wrong places. For the first time in almost forty years, I truly feel loved and accepted, and I know that I am worthy, and that I have purpose.

Feeling loved, accepted, and worthy, I now was able to bring all of my emotions to the surface. Bringing the emotions to the surface, I realized that the negative feelings created labels, and I harbored those negative thoughts for so long. Harboring those negative labels, I was never able to see any other way. Those negative labels had prevented me from living the life that I deserved to have. I had to start identifying the negative labels that I carried. Once I was able to identify the negative labels, I was able to confront them head on in order to free myself. Carrying the negative labels can be so damaging to one's wellbeing. Once I started to see what the labels were doing to my physical body, it became my priority to release the pain and torture. I no longer desire to carry the heavy burdens.

I started attending the classes that my youngest son was going to in order to fulfill his probation requirements. Attending the class, I came to know a very special lady in my life, named the Woo Hoo lady. The Woo Hoo lady is very passionate about what she tries to instill in others when she tries sowing seeds of acceptance. By sowing seeds of acceptance, the goal is to have others see their true purpose in life. In the classes, she does a part where a married couple removes all the negative labels that they have carried around in order to have a healthy marriage. I started watching each week the couple that began removing the labels. Each week the labels that were being removed were different, and by the end of the 8 week session, the couple had removed all of the negative labels in the their life. Watching this couple inspired me to start dealing with the negative labels so that I too could remove them in order to see the greater good in me. Through this couple, I seen myself and it gave me the drive to remove the negative labels.

One day, I began to make a list of the labels that I carried and allowed others to dictate who I truly was. I made a list of the negative labels, as well as the positive labels. The labels are as follows:

Negative Labels
1. Anger
2. Fear
3. Unworthy
4. Unloved
5. Not good enough

6. Always to Blame
7. Something is wrong with me
8. Being mentally ill
9. Selfish
10. No purpose
11. Rejected

Positive Labels
1. Passionate
2. I am loved
3. Caring
4. Appreciated
5. Committed
6. Grateful
7. Worthy
8. Thankful
9. Blessed
10. Not my fault
11. Accepted

Making a list of both negative labels, as well as positive labels helped me see the good in me. The negative labels overpowered me for so long that I was not able to see and feel the good in me. Every time I would tell myself that I was loved and that I was worthy, the negative labels took control. I let the fear of the negative labels control me. Others have seen the good in me; however, I did not believe them because I did not believe in myself. I went through life wondering if I ever had purpose because of what others have done to me and made me feel. Removing the negative labels made me begin to see my purpose in life.

I let the anger of what I went through prevent me from seeing the good in myself. The feeling of being unworthy and unloved prevented me from seeing the real, true, pure love that Jesus and His followers have for me. The feeling of being to blame for everything prevented me from seeing how worthy I really am. The feeling of being unworthy caused many self-esteem issues. I went through life being told I was mentally-ill and that I was bipolar; however, the mental illness that abusers say that I have came from them. I no longer carry the mental illness label because I realized that it was everything that I had been put through. So many of my abusers made me feel selfish because they always told me that I cared only about myself. Because I was always told that, I neglected myself and what my needs were. Now I am able to take care of myself and know that it is ok to take care of myself. Taking care of myself, I have been able to get the proper help needed, and I have been able to start believing in myself and see the positive labels that others see in me.

I now can say that I am a very, passionate, caring, loving, empathetic, trusting, grateful, thankful, blessed child of God who is truly loved, cared for, and nurtured in all of the healthy ways. I now can see my purpose in life, and I can break the cycle. There are times when we get so wrapped up in what we have gone through, that we can't see what we need to in order to better help ourselves. For me, it was the fear of never being accepted and loved that prevented me from seeing this long ago. God does not want us to carry the negative baggage around day after day. God wants us to live each day happy and the way He has planned for us to live. I came to realize that the trauma was not God's fault. Although, God did not do those horrific things to me, He was always there with me in the eye of the storm. God is there for you too, and He is always there for you no matter what the situation is.

Chapter 7 – Breaking the Cycle

Growing up as a child, I grew up with parents that screamed at each other, hit each other, and constantly always hurting one another. They failed to see the torment that they were inflicting upon the kids in the household. I grew up with a man that always came home drunk, waiting to beat me, my brother, or my mother, and always yelling and cussing. What I seen was that my mother tolerated it, and she failed to protect my brother and I. My mother would literally watch the beatings that I received from the drunkard. As I was growing older, I seen this drunkard cheat on my mom so many times; thus, ending in a divorce.

When this drunkard decided to move into his mom's house, my mom constantly worried about what he was doing to the point she would drag my brother and I out in the middle of the night just to see what he was doing. My mom used us kids to get to him, and would literally keep us from him. The pain my mom suffered was inflicted upon us kids. When this drunkard left the home, I lost a part of my mom too. What it seemed was like she didn't see herself surviving from the torment. There was one occasion when my mom allowed us kids to go spend the weekend with our dad. In the middle of the night, our dad received a phone call at 4:00am because my mom was trying to commit suicide. When we arrived at the house, my mom was in the back yard, locked in a running car with her head under the steering wheel.

We immediately called 911 out to the house. We did not have the spare key to the car, so we had to wait until our grandma got there to open the door. While we were waiting, the fire department had searched the house and found some empty medicine bottles. This was very terrifying because we didn't know if my mom was going to remain alive. Our grandma had arrived with the car, so we were able to get her out. The ambulance came and took her to the hospital. I will never forget the robe that my mom was in, and when we got her out of the car, we noticed that my mom had the heat on full blast. To this day, that memory haunts me as if it is happening all over again. Because of that day, I made a promise to myself that I would never ever try to harm myself or anyone else.

After that incident, my mom disappeared for a short while, causing our dad to move back in the home to tend to us kids. Although it was a few months, it felt like an eternity. My mom never called us or ever seen us. Then one day my mom showed up as if everything was ok. I remember the night that she tried getting back with my dad. They got into a big argument and my dad through a telephone and it hit me in the stomach; therefore, going into foster care. Because of the abuse and the instability of my parents, my brother and I had to live with my aunt and uncle. It was a major adjustment to go through because I never knew what was going to happen from that moment on.

Living with my aunt and uncle, my parents had to come there and see us. There were many times my mom always showed up with a different man. That was pretty hurtful to me because I constantly felt that it was a man she desired in her life, and not her kids. I felt ashamed, and I felt like it was my fault because I didn't move when the telephone was thrown. I remember always telling myself that if I had moved out of the way, then I would still be at home. After living with my aunt and uncle for about six months, we were finally able to go back home and live with my mom, but without my dad.

I always remember my mom having multiple men coming in and out of the home. Every time she would see one that I would start getting attached to, they would up and vanish. My mom continued this path until she met her current husband. As far as my dad went, he remarried multiple times. All of my childhood, I had multiple people that came in and out of my life, but no one was permanent. When the people I got attached to left, I was always made to feel that they did not want me; therefore, that was why they left. The family that I had grown up around was not coming around as much; thus making me feel that they did not want me around either.

Coming from a broken home caused me to get into relationships that were the same way I grew up in. At the time, I chased whatever I knew. The friendships and marriages that were unhealthy resulted in what I only knew. What had happened was I went out seeking the parent love that I truly never received. I fell right into disaster because I did not know any better. As I got older, I always promised myself that I would never put my children through anything that I had to go through. Matter of fact, I strived so hard to give them everything that I didn't have growing up.

Although I made a promise to myself, my kids went through some of the same experiences I went through growing up. When I had my daughter, I always hoped that she would not have to endure the kind of sexual abuse that I had to endure throughout life, but it happened. All three of my children suffered the same kind of abuse that I had endured growing up. As a parent, the blame that I carried for so long because I was told it was my fault and that if I hadn't have married who I did it would never have happened. My boys are adults now so they have been able to cope with the best way they can. On the other hand, my daughter is still going through the same thing that I had to go through. When I look into my daughter's eyes, I can see the hurt, pain, and torture that I had to endure throughout life.

My prayer has always been to stop being abused, and to have a loving man that would be a wonderful husband, as well as a loving dad to my children. What I have come to realize is that when I was blessed with a loving man that desires to take care of me the way I am supposed to be cared for, I have let the fear of getting hurt and what I have been through hinder that. The heavy burdens carried for so long has prevented me from accepting the right love in my life. I have went through life being around people that were not true. The type of love they have had for me was conditional, not the type of love Jesus has for me. Once I realized the love that was needed in my life, I was able to remove the labels, break the cycle, and free myself of the pain.

After 41 years of carrying the pain and torture, I now have broken the cycle. Breaking the cycle consisted of freeing myself of my abusers and what they have done, the negative labels I kept bound up, and freeing myself of the brokenness. I am now able to thank God for the bad I had in my life because it showed me how not to be. I have come to a point in my life that I will only accept what is healthy verses what is not healthy. Thank you Jesus for always walking with me and sending the right people needed in my life. I now surround myself around true, pure followers of Jesus.

Chapter 8
Getting Healthy

Growing up without the proper care and nurture and being a single parent, I neglected myself. I am a child of God who puts others' needs before my own. Along the way, I have had some health issues that hindered me throughout life. There were many days where I didn't feel like getting up out of bed, and I began to lose sight of who I was. Losing sight, I began to have self esteem issues that caused me to not see the true beauty within myself. I constantly told myself that maybe if I was pretty, like movie stars, I wouldn't get hurt anymore. When you start losing sight of who you truly are, your mind, heart, and body suffers.

What happens when your mind suffers? When your mind begins to suffer, you start becoming overwhelmed and then depression, anxiety, and post traumatic stress disorder kicks in with great force. This is something that I went through. I constantly buried my past and what happened to me to the point I endured a nervous breakdown. When I went through my nervous breakdown, I felt hopeless, without purpose, like a failure, unloved, and I felt that there was something truly wrong with me. My mind would not shut down because I felt like everything was my fault; thus, losing all faith, hope and belief. Then here came the medicine for depression and anxiety because I had a breakdown. Then I started labeling myself as being mentally ill because that's what others labeled me as. What happens is, the Enemy wants you to to be depressed, anxious, and mentally ill; however, the Enemy is a liar and DO NOT believe him.

After starting counseling and spending time with God, I came to realize that what was wrong with me was not my fault. What I went through was a result of what others have put me through. I'm now at a point in my life where I can truly say "I AM NOT TO BLAME, and IT IS NOT MY FAULT!" No matter what you go through, don't blame yourself because blaming yourself is unhealthy. Getting the proper rest, exercising more, and eating healthier will help your mind.

What happens when your heart suffers? The stress causes great pressure on your heart. When I was twenty-nine, the doctors found two blockages; thus, receiving two cardiac stents. The doctor that was performing the heart catherization said, "I do not know how this girl has not had a double bypass already." The doctors never understood why I had the blockages like I had. Throughout the years, I have had some complications, causing over night hospital stays. A few years ago, the doctor found another blockage. The blockage was only at thirty percent, so I did not need another cardiac stent. Although the doctors never understood the blockages I had, I knew. Stress is what caused the blockages, and stress causes severe chest pains. After much prayer over my third blockage and eliminating stress in my life, my recent cardiac testing shows no blockage. God's hands were at work.

There are great rewards when you eliminate the stress in your life, exercise regularly, and eat healthier. Eating a heart healthy diet can lower your chances of getting plaque build up in your arteries. There are great rewards when removing the stressors in your life because stress is the number one killer, and stress causes your heart to work harder. Walking daily is very healthy for your heart. I love my daily walks because I spend time with God, clearing my mind. I always have a special friend that walks with me, Jesus. There is no greater joy than knowing Jesus walks beside me every step I take. Not only does He do this with me, He does it for all. Not only does He walk with me, He talks with me along the way. I thank Jesus every day for always being my true, special, friend.

What happens when your body suffers? Carrying the pain and burdens for so long caused great pain to my body. To hide from the pain, I constantly stayed on the go, never slowing down. I always told myself that I was like the energizer bunny who kept going, and going, and going. One would think that the energizer bunny could go on forever; however, the bunny needs recharged too. I went through life doing everything on my own because I was never dependent on others getting me through life. Being a single mom of three, I worked two jobs at times just to make ends meet. Sitting down was never a part of my daily routine, unless I was driving, eating, or attending church. By not slowing down and relaxing, I put too much stress on my body. Pushing my body to the max, I would constantly hurt because I kept pushing my body too hard. What I have come to realize is that when you over stress your body, you have to slow down and rest more often. My boys have always told me to slow down, but I was too stubborn to listen. What I realize is that it is ok to slow down and rest your body. I am never alone, and I let my faith in God carry me through.

Ridding myself of stress, there have been things that I have done that has greatly helped me. The following list are tools that I used to help myself, and the list is as follows:

1. Journaling
2. Reading self -help books
3. Listening to music and getting into the lyrics
4. Decorating my house full of inspiration
5. Daily walks with Jesus
6. Working in the yard
7. Ridding myself of artificial flowers
8. Eating healthier
9. Christian counseling
10. Surrounding myself with true followers of Christ
11. Bible studies
12. Support groups
13. Doing something for myself on a daily basis
14. Turning my phone off at night, and not answering every call or text.
15. Laughing and smiling because it is the best medicine.

Getting healthy is ok to do because in the long run you will become stronger. Don't let what others have done to you control your mind and heart or body. Let God be your Healer because He is the Mighty Physician. Whatever you may go through, never lose sight of yourself, and always remember to take care of yourself. You are the only one that can take care of yourself because no body else will. Always remember to laugh and smile because you are truly loved. You are beautiful, and always let your light shine. No matter the hurt, the pain, or the bruises, the cross made you flawless. Tell yourself that you can and that you will. No matter the bumps or how deep the wounds are, always find grace in God.

Chapter 9
Believing in Yourself

Growing up, I lacked the belief in myself because no one else believed in me. Everything I tried to do in life left me feeling that it was never good enough for anyone. I spent too much time trying to live by what others wanted me to. I lived by my emotions and how others told me to live. I figured if I did that, then they would love me and accept me. As time went on, I asked myself "Who are you truly living your life for? Is it yourself? Is it others? Is it God?" The reality was that I was living for everyone else.

Living for others led to being controlled by all the artificial flowers, also known as relationships, I had in my life. The relationships I had most of my life I call artificial flowers because artificial flowers are fake, and artificial flowers can't grow. When artificial flowers get watered, they still can not grow. It takes a little rain to make love grow, as well as, planting seeds. Realizing that I was being controlled by relationships that prevented me from growing, I decided to start pulling the fake flowers out of my garden, my life. Even if it was just one at a time, it was helping me believe in myself. By weeding them out, my abusers were beginning to lose control over me.

There was a time in my life I lost everything I worked so hard for in life. Once again, I became shattered, destroyed, and angry because my abusers were controlling me once again. This time my abusers started using other people to control me to. This time I was all alone trying to fight an army by myself. I lost the fight within me because I did not have an army of my own to help me. Being controlled by the abusive army, I sold my home on false promises, I lost my job from the harassment, and I lost my car because it got vandalized to the point that I could not drive it. No matter how hard the war was to fight, I still managed to pick up the pieces in order to survive. It didn't matter where I went or what I did, I was constantly being tortured by the war, and the abusers that were battling the war.

At this point in my life, I gave up on myself, and I lost all hope. I started blaming myself, as well as God. I started believing that my purpose in life was to be battered, torn, and beaten all my life. Matter of fact, I felt like I was a burden to everyone else. All that I did was cry every day, while praying for those that had wronged me. I isolated myself because I did not feel worthy enough. I felt like a nobody. I rejected my friends because I did not feel special enough to be around. The only thing I could do and continue to do, was pray for a miracle.

Praying for a miracle, God woke me up and started showing me that I was truly a beautiful child of His, from the inside to the outside. God placed one of His children in my path to start showing me the true beauty, all through his kind words. My special, brother in Christ, started helping me see the good in me. God worked through him to show me that I am special, kind, loving, beautiful, and that I am more than good enough. No matter what I have went through or what I go through now, God uses His children to reach me when I am at my lowest. God has truly blessed me with my brother because my brother gave me the inspiration to start blossoming. I became inspired to turn away from the broken girl and blossom into a real flower. Through God's hands, I started believing in myself. I had to open up my heart enough to allow God to show me what I was never able to see from the start.

There can be true miracles that happen in your life when you truly believe. Sometimes hope can be frail; thus destroying your belief. You will never know what miracles that YOU can truly achieve until you start believing. Praying to God and seeking faith is what you can do to start believing in the miracles that He has in store for you. Never let others control you to the point you quit believing in yourself. When you start believing in yourself, you become half way there. When battling wars, let God and His children be your army. Take up the shield of faith, and keep it close to your heart. May God bless you today and always. Tell yourself that you can and that you will achieve any obstacle that may come your way.

Chapter 10
The Victory: Becoming a Survivor

For quite some time, I was always afraid to talk about what has happened to me out of fear of what would happen to me. Throughout life, I have been threatened and made to feel that no one would listen. The things that abusers threaten us with can be very damaging. I used the fear as a way to isolate myself, stop me from getting help, and not taking proper care of myself. When we go through traumatic times in life, we instantly become afraid. Although, we get told it's not ok to tell, we often don't tell out of fear of not being believed or what harm may come our way. I can remember when I first started telling my mom what her husband was doing to me. She did not believe me because she lives a life of denial. I was told that I was a liar, and that those things never happened. To this day, my mom protects her husband. Now that I am older and can make my own decisions, I have chosen to put great distance between them and myself.

There were things that I was threatened that would happen to me if I told anyone. For the longest time, I was so scared that I never told the truth, and I kept the truth bottled up for so long. Matter of fact, I hid behind the truth. I began living a life that was not real; thus, living with fake self. The person I was having to be was very miserable. I cried all the time. I remained battered, torn, and tossed by my abusers. I had to endure so much pain because I always was made to feel that I had to protect the guilty ones. It took many years to start speaking out, and I used my faith in God to be my comfort because He is the Great Comforter. I started letting the truth out because the truth will set you free; therefore, I quit letting others control me and my emotions. At this point in my life, I will never hide behind the truth. God is truth and the whole truth. There is never a need to live behind the truth, and no matter if we feel that we will never be listened to, God listens and God knows. God gives us the courage we need to come forward, and God is our voice when no one will listen.

Throughout life, I allowed fear to take hold of me and bind me in chains. It did not matter what the situation was, fear always controlled me. There were so many times in my life that I ran from situations out of fear of being hurt, being alone, feeling ashamed, and feeling that I would never amount to much. What I had to start doing was start confronting my fears one by one. It did not matter what the fear was or is, I started overcoming my fears. It did not matter how small the fear was or how big the fear was, I started confronting the fears. Because fear was controlling my life, I was not living by faith. I now am letting faith in God guide me, not letting fear control me because fear is a liar. Zach Williams could not sing it any better when he sings:

> "Fear, He is a liar
> He Will take your breath
> Stop you in your steps
> Fear he is liar
> He will rob your rest
> Steal your happiness
> Cast your fear in the fire
> Cause fear he is a liar."

There were things in my life that I had to rid myself from in order to reach the victory. I had to get rid of the insecurities in order to be confident in myself. Lack of confidence in one's self is a terrible way to live, and God wants you to be confident in your ability in Him. I had to rid myself with the idea of always trying to obtain the approval from others. When you put your faith in trying to win the approval by man, instead of God, it opens up your life for disappointment, as well as, a world of failed expectations. I had to quit blaming myself. We cannot control circumstances, but we can control our reactions to the circumstance. Most importantly, I had to quit living by fear. When we operate in fear, we essentially defect our original design and function. We were all created in God's image, and God created us to live a life of love and serving others. Living in fear causes you to live a life that is closed; thus, causing us to be only concerned about our survival. This is not God's will for His children. I had to cast my fears down, leave them at Jesus's feet, and pick them up no more. By laying everything down at Jesus's feet, I no longer am a victim. By God's Grace, I made it to victory. I AM A SURVIVOR. Now that I become a survivor, God has been blessing me each and every day, and He will continue to bless me.

Becoming a survivor is the most precious thing. In order for true, divine healing to be done, you must move to the victory side. When you free yourself of the dead weight, you open yourself for big blessings. I promise you that when you become a survivor, YOU will be blessed in ways that you may not see. God will make a way for you. God will open up new doors for you; however, old doors must be shut first. He will never close one door without opening up a new one. Let faith and trust in the Lord be your guide. Always remember, if He has done this for me, He will do it for YOU. Let this true living testimony bless you today, tomorrow, and always. Keep on shining and smiling because YOU ARE TRULY LOVED. God loves you, and so do I. Always remember that God promised us healing, and God is a God of promises. God will never break his promises that He has promised His children.

Dear Heavenly Father,

"Happy Father's Day. Thank you for being the Father that I have needed in my life. Thank you for what you have done for me, as well as others. Thank you for loving me enough that you sent your Son so that I could be washed away from my sins. Thank you for taking all the pain away, and thank you for making my heart brand new. YOU are the reason this book was written, so today I gift this book to you on this very special Father's Day. Father, I thank you for all of the good in my life, as well as the bad. Thank you for allowing me to be a blessing to others, and allowing me to continue to be a blessing. I lift up those that don't know you Father, and I pray that this special gift that I have given to you today will touch the lives of those who are broken and lost. I pray for each and every reader of this book. I pray that you take your gift and share it with the world and reach the broken and lost so that they can come to know you, just as I did. I LOVE YOU. In Jesus's sweet and holy name, AMEN."

JENNEFER PADDOCK

Poems

Poems that gave me the inspiration to never give up.
(This section is dedicated to Darin "Tadpole" Davis. Thank you brother for all the sweet words that God laid on your heart. YOU are and will always be a true blessing in my life.)

Walking Through Life's Struggles

I remember walking through life
And the struggles and strife.
On the outside all smiles, but
On the inside the pain unbearable.
Just going through the motions

Looking for that secret potion.
Same routines day after day,
Going on what seemed my merry way.

Then I realized I was in need
My heart and soul to be freed.
That night, I hit my knees,
Begging God "please, oh please."

Give me strength I need
To open my eyes to a new day.
Then God reached down and put
His arms all around me saying,
"My child, all you had to do was ask. I am willing and able."

One day my life was changed
In an instant, blink of an eye
I will always remember the struggles and strife.

So my advice to you
Never forget where you came from
And where you are going
Or who brought you through life's struggles.

JENNEFER PADDOCK

Thanks For Making Me a Better Person

I love you , Not only for what you are,
But what I am because of YOU
I love you for not only what you have become,
But for how you changed me

I love you because you have done
More than any creed could have done
And more than fate could have done

I love you because you have made me who I am today
When you waltzed back into my life

One Day

One day there was a broken girl
Who was just going through the motions
She had buried the pain down deep
Night after night not getting sleep

Never knowing how truly blessed she was
Because she was burdened by all the stresses
But one night she hit her knees
Asking God to send a sign
That would open her eyes and bring about a change

The fog was lifted
The pain was gone
She began to sing a new song
Her smile reappeared
And her personality brightened

One day there was a girl
Who blossomed into a beautiful flower
Thank you Jesus for never giving up on me.

JENNEFER PADDOCK

Magic Wand

I wish I had a magic wand
To make it go away;
I'd wave my scepter over you
Until you were okay.

I'd think good thoughts;
I'd send you love;
I'd transmit healing vibes; My word and I would surely beat
Whatever the doctor prescribes.

But there is no magic scepter, so
I cannot cast a spell;
Just know you've often in my thoughts,
And I hope you'll soon be well.

Here For You

When you're sad and depressed
I will be here to put a smile on your face
To tell you how beautiful you are

When you are angry and frustrated
I will be here to calm you down

When you're hurt and in tears
I will be here to dry your eyes and ease your pain

When you are lonely
I will be here to comfort you

When you feel unloved
I will tell you how important you are

When you are full of worry
I will be here to worry with you

I promise, I will always be here for you!!

JENNEFER PADDOCK

A Special Friend

A friend like you is hard to find
Precious like a diamond
With your sparkling smile

Always with a warming touch
And knowing just what to say
Friend's crying always heard

So with all my heart I say
Just what you mean to me
As another season begins

I hope your days are filled with love
And your dream/wishes fulfilled
May God hold you in his gentle embrace

You are important to me my special friend
So forever you will be in my heart
May God always bless you

Never Stop Smiling

You smile on the outside
Yet cry on the inside
When you smile
It is just your way to hide
Your many hurts, so obvious to me

You laugh the hurt…You are
Wiping away your tears…You are
You smile to forget your fears, I know

I want to hold you til all the pains bleed away
I want to see you smile til you no longer cry

You scream on the inside…I know
Craving for a healthy touch
You can soak in more…Trust me
I will be here even when your pain goes away

I will always love you,
So don't ever stop smiling

JENNEFER PADDOCK

Breathe

In my very weakness
I humbly kneel before your cross
In desperation I fearfully seek
You and You alone
I have found no other
Who is able to restore my soul
Won't you make me whole

Breathe on, breathe on me
God please come and transform me
You and You alone are all I need
Power of God breathe on me

I'm ready to take up my cross
And live for you daily
No matter what I have to surrender
Reveal what you would have of me
Cleanse me from all my sins
Use me now for your glory

God's Promise to Us

I make this solemn promise to you that
I will love you when you need to be loved,
Your doctor when you are ill,
Your army when you go to war
Your umbrella when life rains down on you
Your rock when you get weary
Your shield when you need defense
Your spirit when you are drained
Your pillow when you need rest
Your voice when no one can hear you
Your ear when no one will listen
Your comfort when you feel pain
Your hero when you are under duress
Your sunshine when darkness fails
Your answer when questions arise
Your inspiration to overcome obstacles
Your hand to hold when you are frightened

I am yours…All of me!!!

Songs

Songs that always gave me hope and belief when going through the storms in life. (This section is dedicated to the singers that allows God to work through them with all the kind, precious, sweet lyrics. Thank you for allowing God to work through you. YOU are a true blessing.)

BY GOD'S GRACE: A TRUE LIVING TESTIMONY

Broken Girl
By: Matthew West

"Look what he he's done to you
It isn't fair
Your light was bright and new
But he didn't care
He took the heart of a little girl
And made it grow up to fast

Now words like innocence
Don't mean anything
You hear the music play
But you can't sing
Those pictures in your mind
Keep you locked up inside…your past

This is a song for the broken girl
The one pushed aside by the cold, cold world
You are
Hear me when I say
You're not the worthless they made you feel
There is a love they can never steal away
And you don't have to stay the broken girl

Those damaged goods you see
In your reflection
Love sees them differently
Love sees perfection
A beautiful display
Of healing on the way tonight"

JENNEFER PADDOCK

He Touched Me
By: Gaither Vocal Band

"Shackled by a heavy burden
'Neath a load of guilt and shame
Then the hand of Jesus touched me
And now I am no longer the same

He touched me, oh He touched me
And oh the joy that floods my soul
Something happened and Now I know
He touched me and made me whole

Since I met this blessed Savior
Since He's cleansed and made me whole
Oh I will never cease to praise Him
I'll shout it while eternity rolls

He touched me, oh He touched
And oh the joy that floods my soul
Something happened and Now I know
He touched me and made me whole."

BY GOD'S GRACE: A TRUE LIVING TESTIMONY

Amazing Grace
By: Susan Broyle

"Amazing Grace, How sweet the sound
That saved a wretch like me
I once was lost, but now I am found
Was blind, but now I see

Through many dangers, toils, and snares
I have already come
Tis grace that brought me safe thus far
And grace will lead me home

The Lord hath promised good to me,
His word my hope secures.
He will my shield and portion me
As long as life endures.

When we have been there ten thousand years
Bright, shining as the sun
We've no less days to sing God's praise
Than when we first begun."

JENNEFER PADDOCK

More Than Anything
By" Natalie Grant

"I know if you wanted to you could wave your hand
Spare me this heartache, and change Your plan
And I know any second you could take my pain away
But even if you don't, I pray

Help me want the Healer, more than healing
Help me want the Savior, more than saving
Help me want the Giver, more than the giving
Oh help me want you Jesus, more than anything

You know that my faith is weak
And you know that I'd give anything for a remedy
And I'll ask a thousand more times to set me free today
Oh but even if you don't, I pray

Help me want the Healer, more than healing
Help me want the Savior, more than saving
Help me want the Giver, more than the giving
Oh help me want you Jesus, more than anything

When I am desperate and my heart's overcome
All that I need, You've already done
When I am desperate and my heart's overcome
All that I need, you've already done
Oh Jesus
Help me want you more, than anything"

The Climb
By: Miley Cyrus

"I can almost see it, The dream I'm dreaming but
There's a voice inside my head saying, You'll never reach,
Every step I'm taking, Every move I make feels
Lost with no direction
My faith is shaking but I
Gotta keep trying, Gotta keep my head held high

There's always gonna be another mountain
I'm always gonna wanna make it move
Always gonna be an uphill battle
Sometimes I'm gonna have to lose
Ain't about how fast I get there
Ain't about what's waiting on the other side, It's the climb

The struggles I'm facing, The chances I'm taking
Sometimes might knock me down but, No I'm not breaking
I may not know it, But these are the moments that
I'm going to remember most yeah, Just got to keep going
And I, I gotta be strong, Just keep pushing on, 'cause

There's always gonna be another mountain
I'm always gonna wanna make it move
Always gonna be an uphill battle
Sometimes I'm gonna have to lose
Ain't about how fast I get there
Ain't about what's waiting on the other side, it's the climb"

JENNEFER PADDOCK

You're Going to Be Ok
By: Brian and Jen Johnson

"I know it's all you've got to just, be strong
And it's a fight just to keep it together, together
I know you think, that you care too far gone
But hope is never lost
Hope is never lost

Hold on, don't let go
Hold on, don't let go

Just take one step closer
Put one foot in front of the other
You'll get through this
Just follow the light in the darkness
You're gonna be ok

I know your heart is heavy from those nights
Just remember that you're a fighter, a fighter
You never know just what tomorrow holds
And you're stronger than you know
Stronger than you know

Just take one step closer
Put one foot in front of the other
You'll get through this
Just follow the light in the darkness
You're gonna be ok

And when the night is closing in
Don't give up and don't give in
This won't last, it's not the end. It's not the end

You're gonna be ok
When the night is closing in
Don't give up and don't give in"

JENNEFER PADDOCK

Chain Breaker
By: Zach Williams

"If you've been walking the same old road for miles and miles
If you've been hearing the same old voice tell the same old lies
If you're trying to feel the same old holes inside
There's a better life
There's a better life

If you've got pain
He's a pain taker
If you feel lost
He's a way maker
If you need freedom or saving
He's a prison-shaking Savior
If you've got chains
He's a chain breaker

We've all search for the light of day in the dead of night
We've all found ourselves worn out from the same old fight
We've all run to things we know just ain't right
And there's a better life
There's a better life

If you've got pain
He's a pain taker
If you feel lost
He's a way maker
If you need freedom or saving
He's a prison-shaking Savior
If you've got chains
He's a chain breaker"

Different
By: Micha Tyler

"I don't wanna hear anymore, teach me to listen
I don't wanna see anymore, give me a vision
That you could move this heart, to be set apart
I don't need to recognize the man in the mirror
And I don't wanna trade Your plan, for something familiar
I can't waste a day, I can't stay the same

I wanna be different
I wanna be changed
Till all of me is gone
And all that remains
Is a fire so bright
The whole world can see
That there's something different
So come and be different In me

And I don't wanna spend my life, stuck in a pattern
And I don't wanna gain this world but lose what matters
And I'm giving up, everything because

I wanna be different
I wanna be changed
Till all of me is gone
And all that remains
Is a fire so bright
The whole world can see
That there's something different
So come and be different; oh-oh
Continued On Next Page

JENNEFER PADDOCK

I know that I am far, from perfect
But through you, the cross still says, I'm worth it
So take this beating in my heart and
Come and finish what You started
When they see me, let them see You
Cause I wanna be different

I wanna be different
I wanna be changed
Till all of me is gone
And all that remains
Is a fire so bright
The whole world can see
That there's something different
So come and be different
I just wanna be different
So could You be different
In me?"

BY GOD'S GRACE: A TRUE LIVING TESTIMONY

Fear is a Liar
By: Zach Williams

When he told you you're not good enough
When he told you you're not right
When he told you you're not strong enough
To put up a good fight
When he told you you're not worthy
When he told you you're not loved
When he told you you're not beautiful
That you'll never be enough

Fear, He is a liar
He Will take your breath
Stop you in your steps
Fear he is liar

He will rob your rest
Steal your happiness
Cast your fear in the fire
Cause fear he is a liar.

When he told you were troubled
You'll forever be alone
When he told you you should run away
You'll never find a home
When he told you you were dirty
And you should be ashamed
When he told you you could be the one
That grace could never change
Continued On Next Page

JENNEFER PADDOCK

Fear, He is a liar
He Will take your breath
Stop you in your steps
Fear he is liar
He will rob your rest
Steal your happiness
Cast your fear in the fire
Cause fear he is a liar"

BY GOD'S GRACE: A TRUE LIVING TESTIMONY

Eye of the Storm
By Ryan Stevenson

"In the eye of the storm
You remain in control
And in the middle of the war
You guard my soul
You alone are the anchor
When my sails are torn
Your love surrounds me
In the eye of the storm

When the solid ground is falling out from underneath my feet
Between the black skies, and my red eyes, I can barely see
When I realize I've been sold out by my friends and my family
I can feel the rain reminding me
In the eye of the storm, You remain in control
In the middle of the war, You guard my soul
You alone are the anchor, when my sails are torn
Your love surrounds me
In the eye of the storm

When my hopes and dreams are far from me
And I'm running out of faith
I see the future I picture slowly fade away
And when the tears of pain and heartache
Are pouring down my face
I find my peace in Jesus's name
Continued On Next Page

JENNEFER PADDOCK

In the eye of the storm
You remain in control
And in the middle of the war
You guard my soul
You alone are the anchor
When my sails are torn
Your love surrounds me
In the eye of the storm

When the tests come in and the doctors says
I've only got a few months left
It's like a bitter pill I'm swallowing
I can barely breath
And when addiction steals my baby girl
And there's nothing I can do
My only hope is to trust You
I trust You, Lord

The lord is my Shepherd
I have all that I need
He let's me rest in green meadows
He leads me beside peaceful streams
He renews my strength
He guides me along right paths, bringing honor to His name
Even when I walk through the darkest valley, I will not be afraid
For you are close beside me"

BY GOD'S GRACE: A TRUE LIVING TESTIMONY

JENNEFER PADDOCK

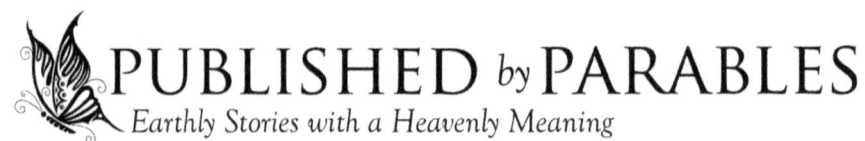

www.ingramcontent.com/pod-product-compliance
Lightning Source LLC
Chambersburg PA
CBHW060032040426
42333CB00042B/2400